MY FRUIT BOOK

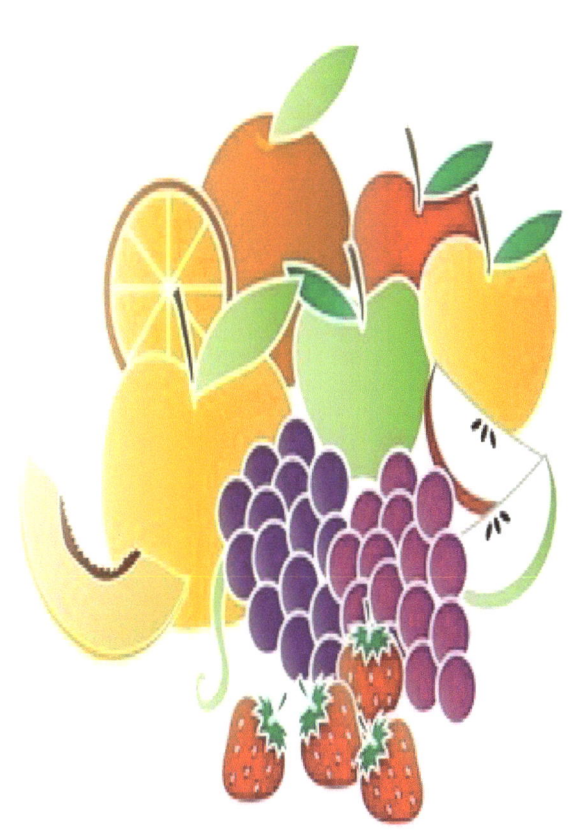

WRITTEN BY: MELISSA L. BRYANT

I dedicate this book to my children Lavicia, Vyshonn, Damarius, Darrell and Rashad, who I love so much.
 I dedicate this book to my nieces Kyrenne and Claudia. I dedicate this book to my nephews James, Conner and Amarie.
I dedicate this book to all the children at Daleville Christian Fellowship and the children around the world.
Thank you all for the Love and support. God bless you all and the best is yet to come.

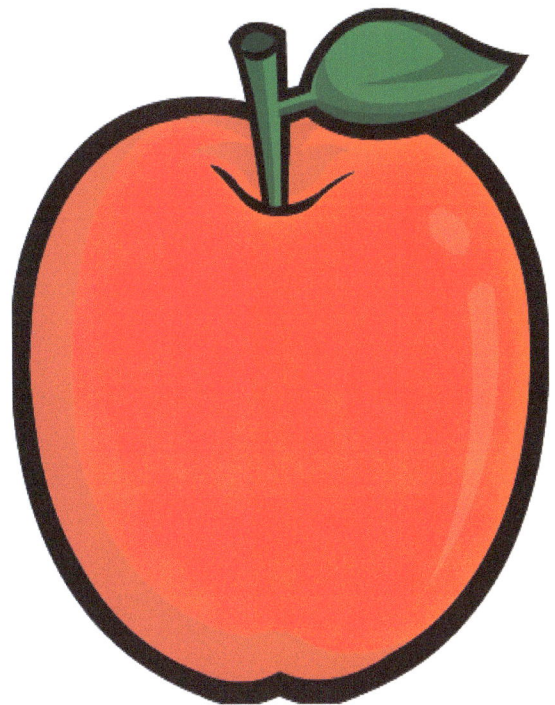

I like red apple. What about you?

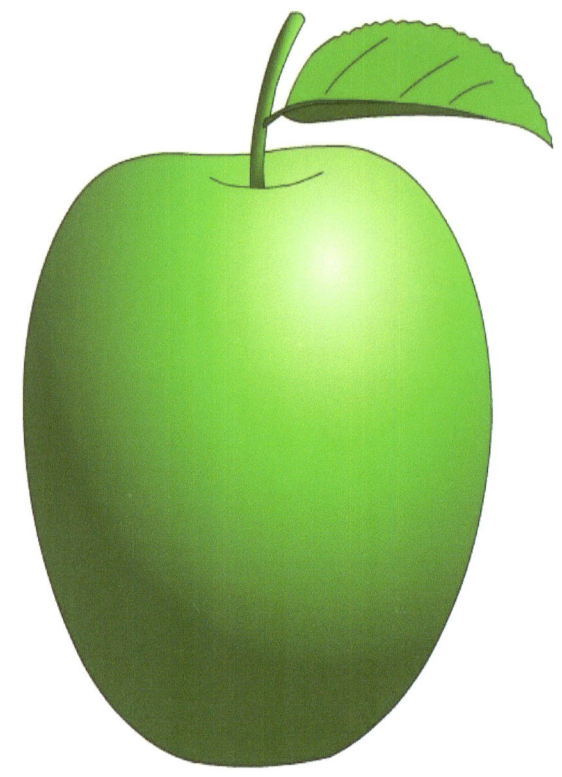

I love green apple. What about you?

I like to eat a peach. What about you?

I love oranges. What about you?

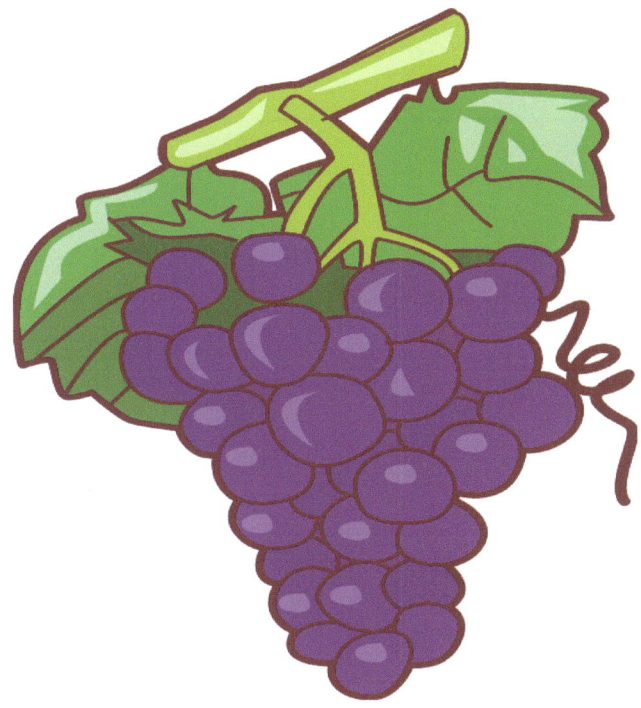

I like grapes. What about you?

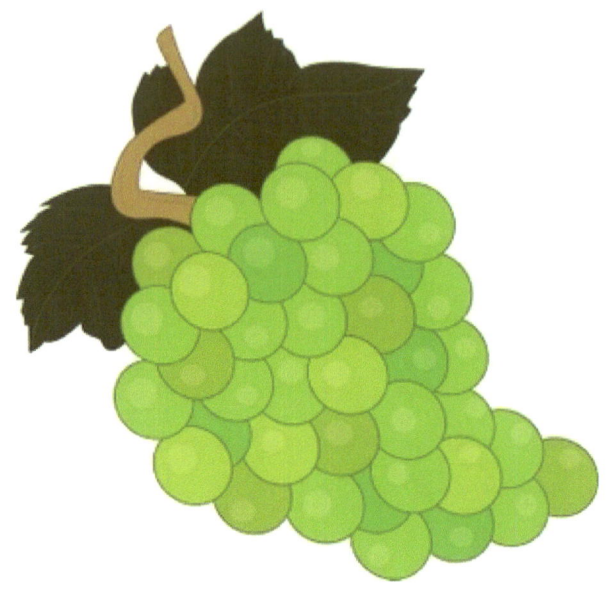

I love green grapes. What about you?

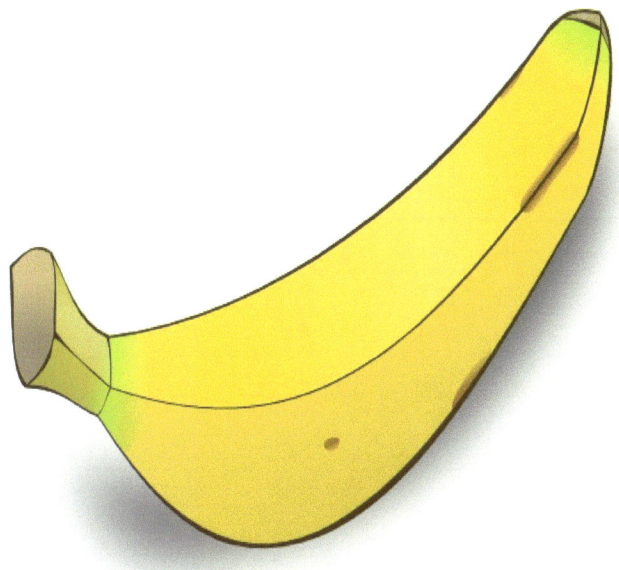

I like banana. What about you?

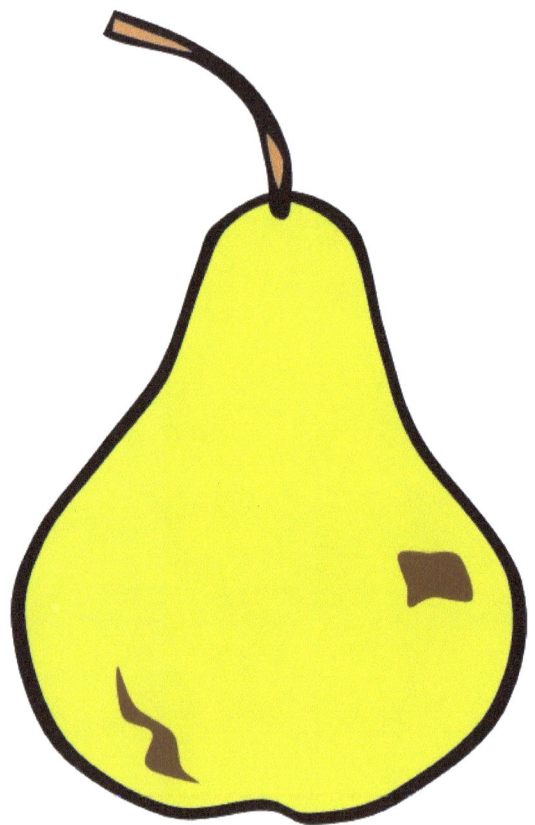

I like pears. What about you?

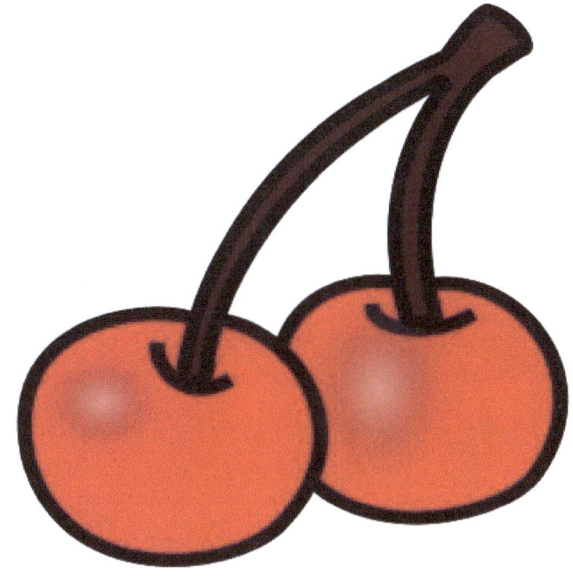

I like cherries. What about you?

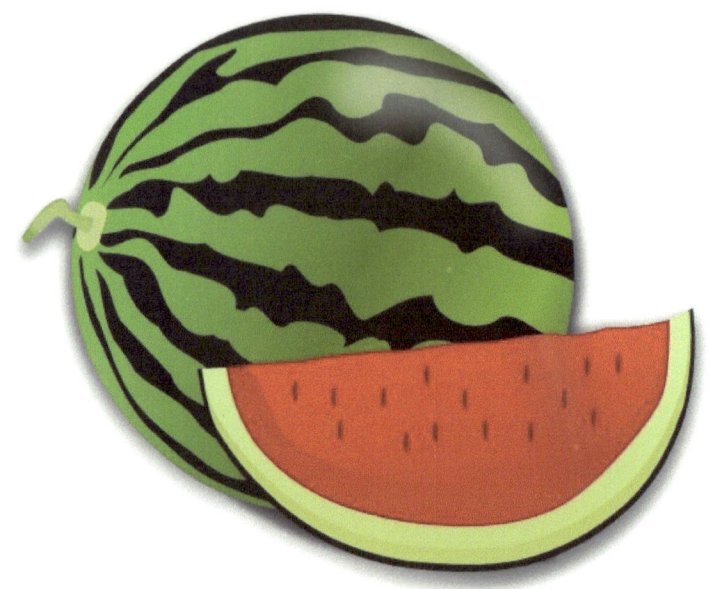

I like watermelon. What about you?

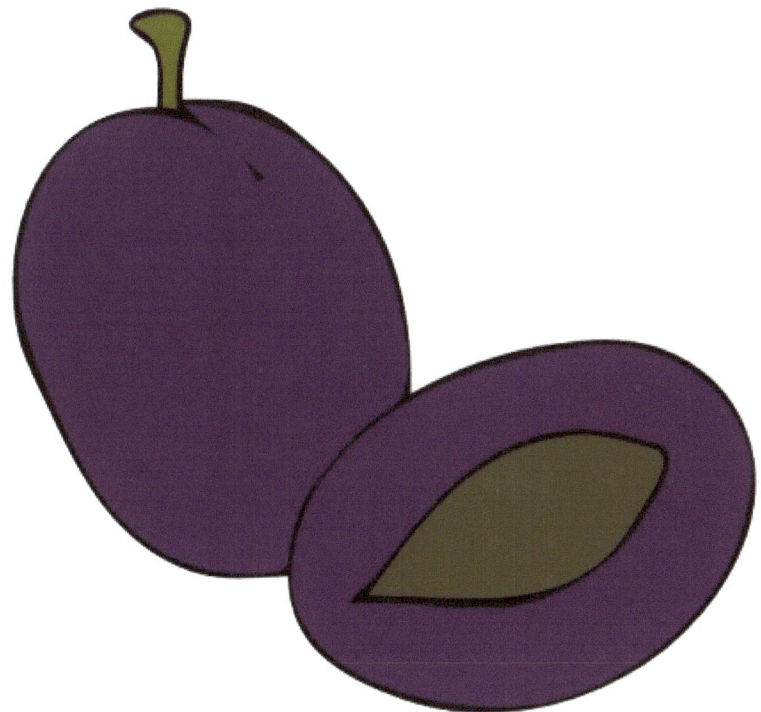

I like plums. What about you?

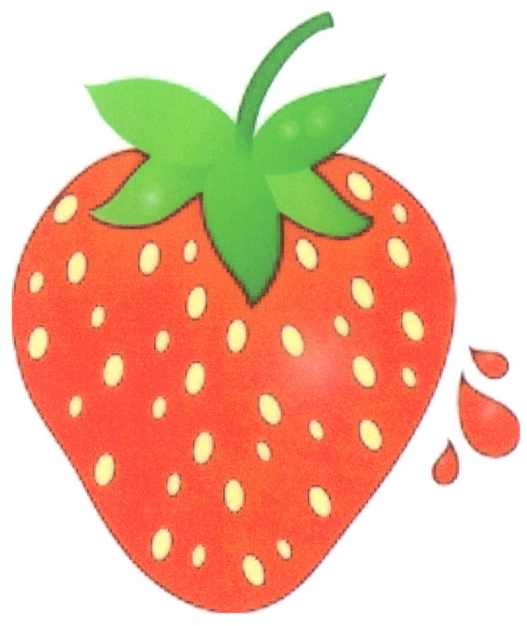

I like strawberry. What about you?

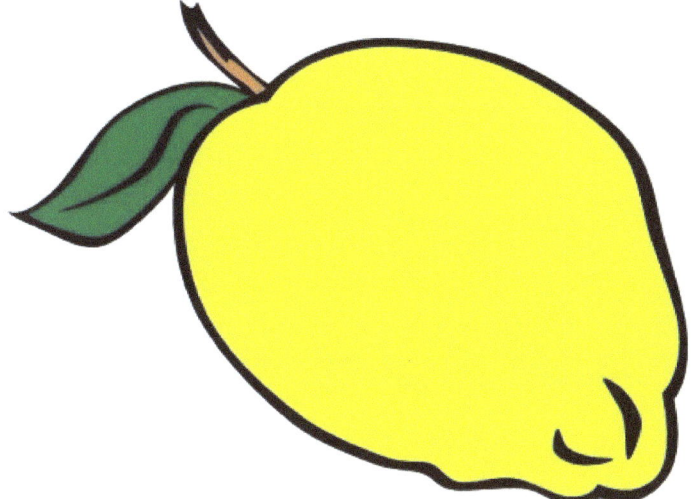

I like lemon. What about you?

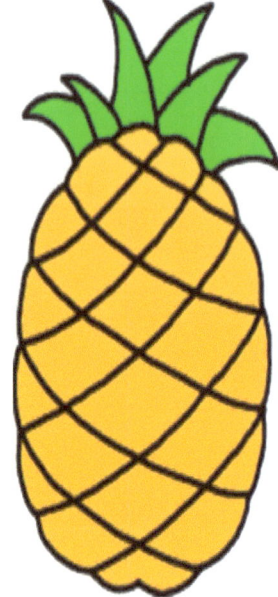

I like pineapples. What about you?

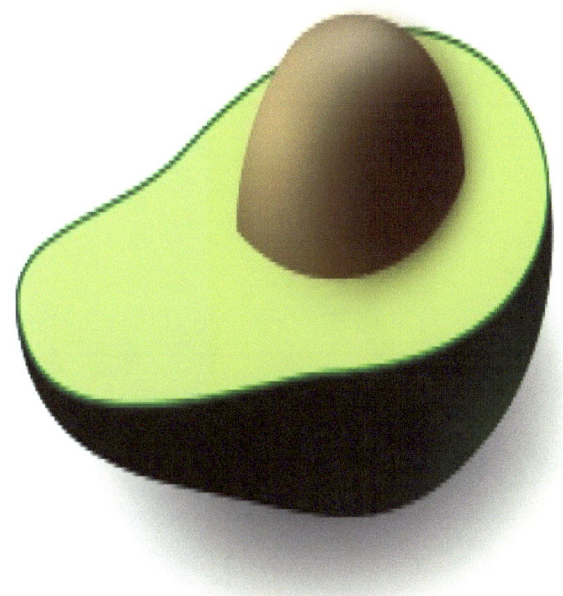

I like avocado. What about you?

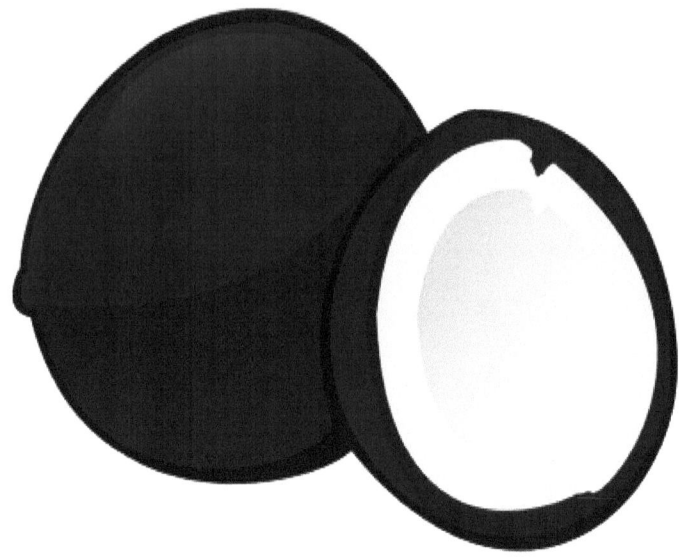

I like coconut. What about you?

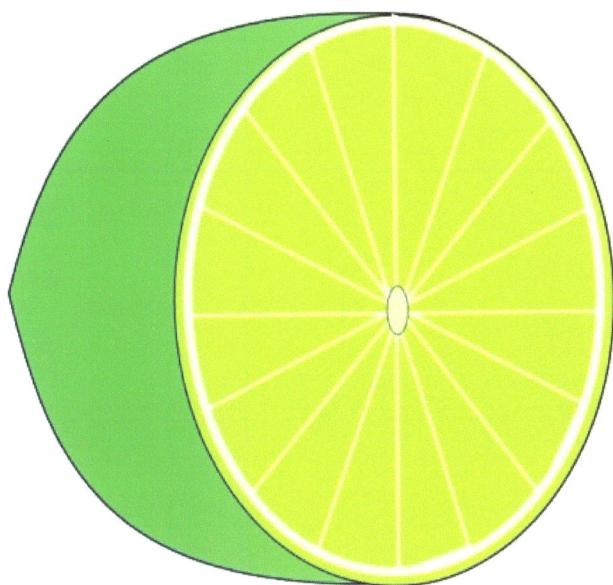

I like lemon lime. What about you?

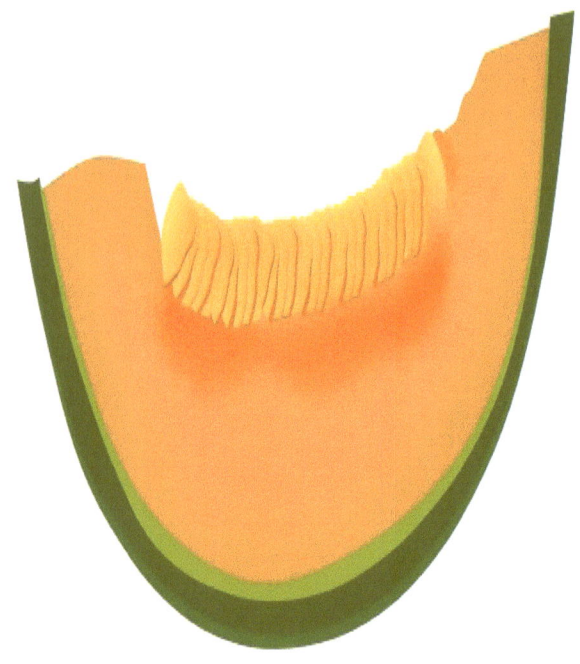

I like cantaloupe. What about you?

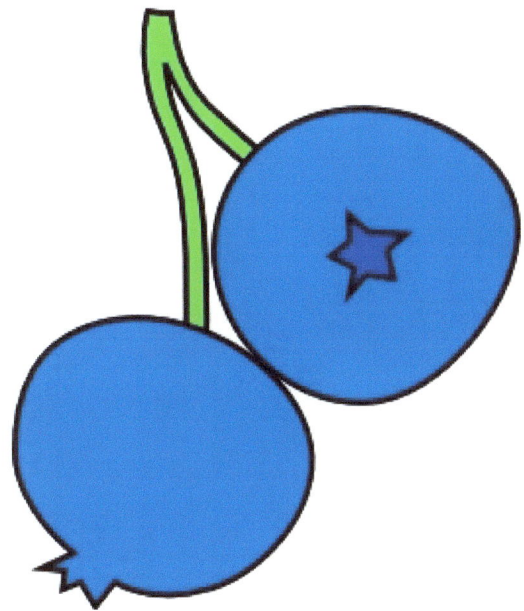

I like blueberries. What about you?

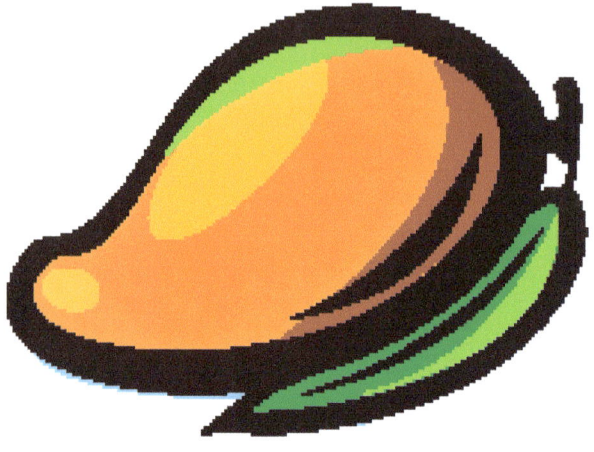

I like mango. What about you?

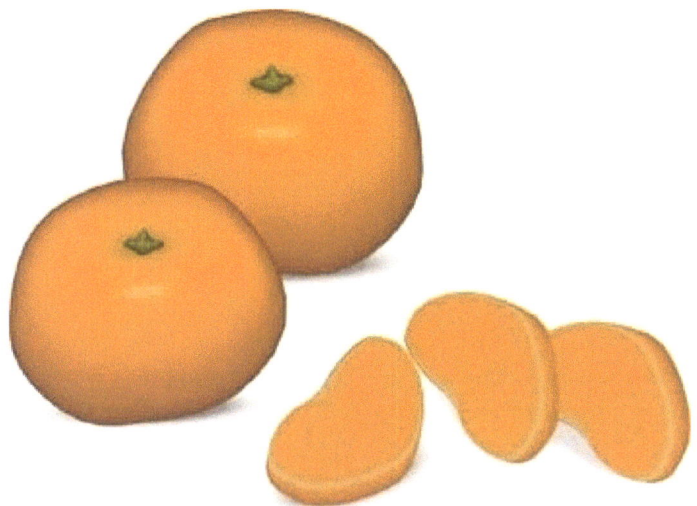

I like mandarin oranges. What about you?

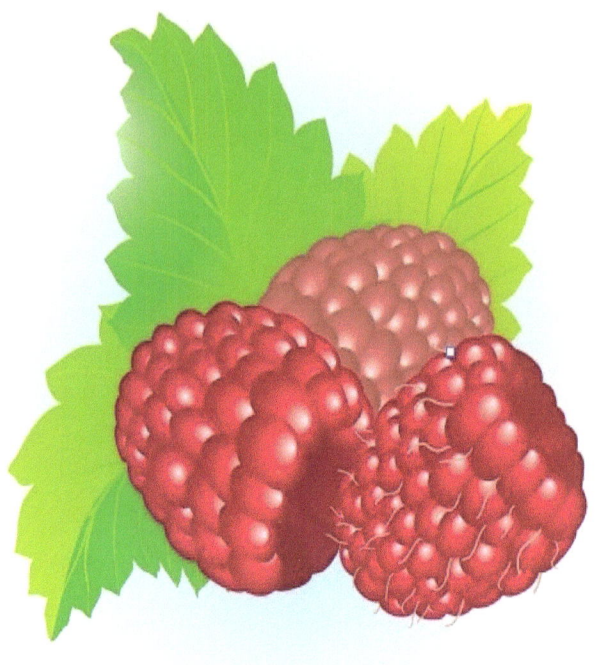

I like raspberries. What about you?

I like tangerine. What about you?

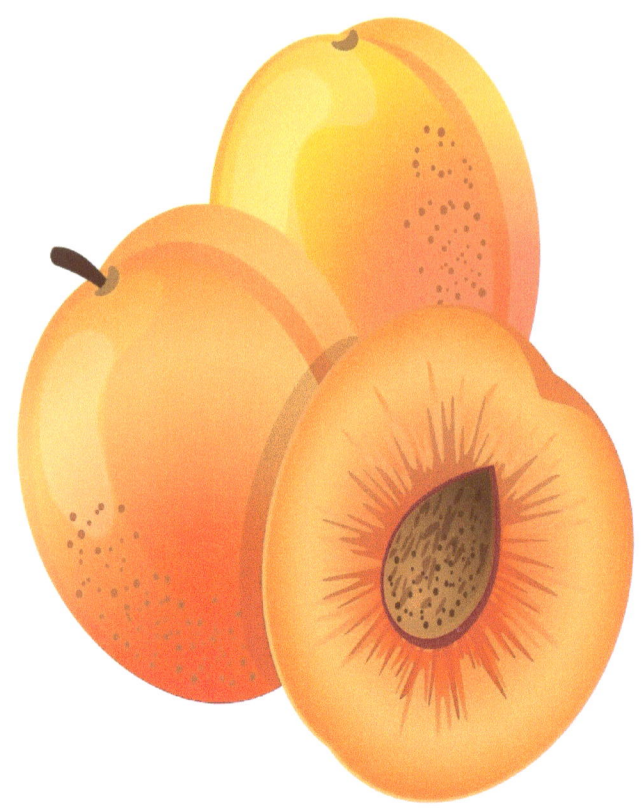

I like apricot. What about you?

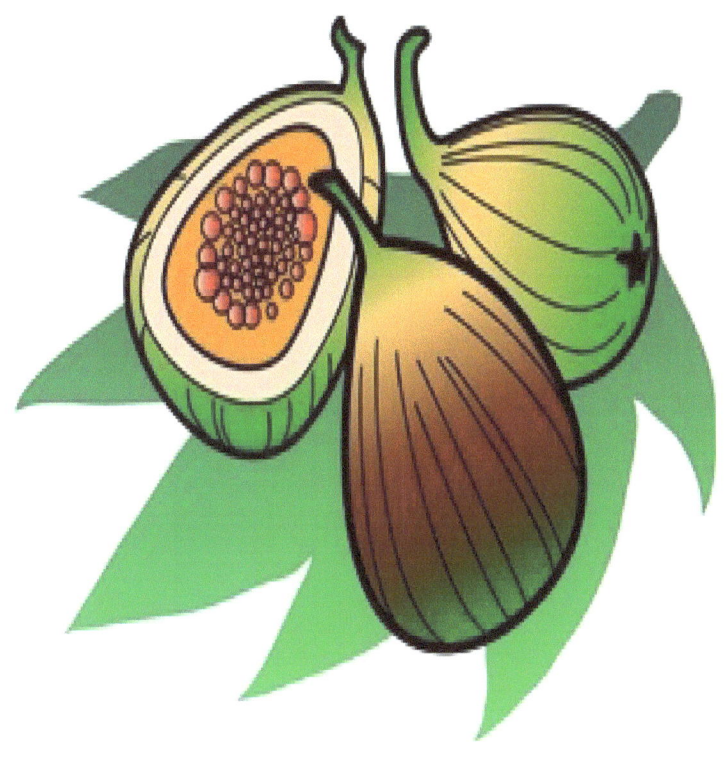

I like figs. What about you?

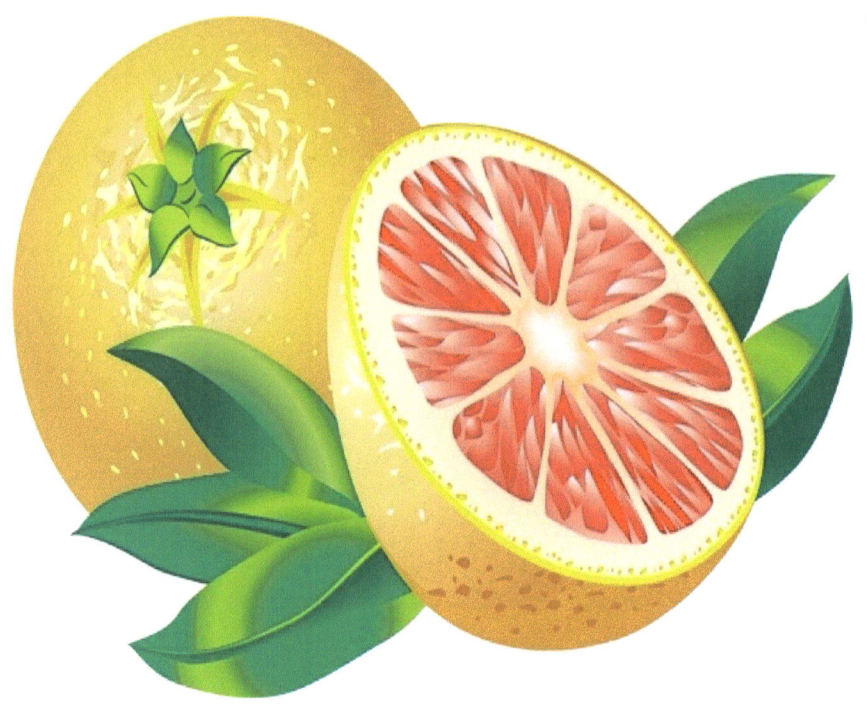

I love pink grapefruits. What about you?

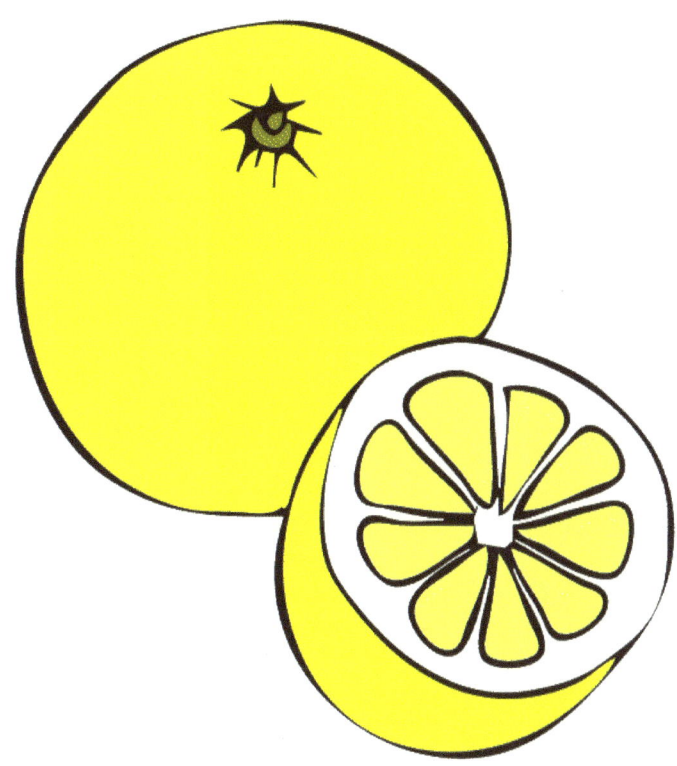

I like grapefruits. What about you?

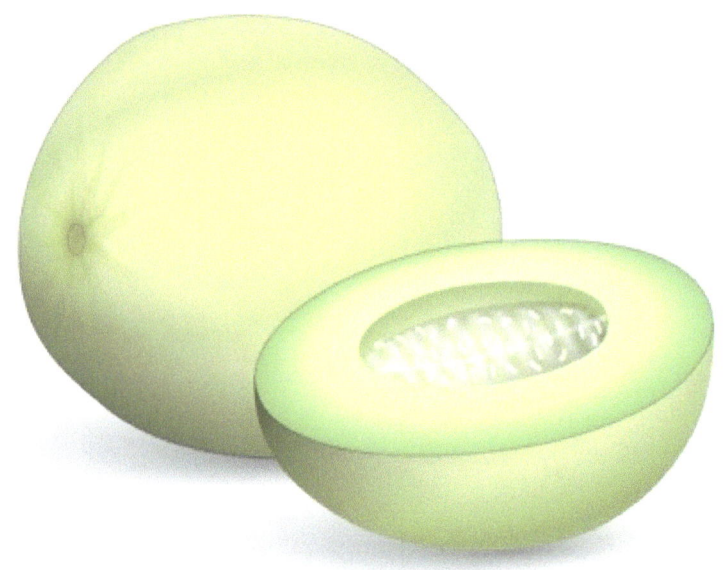

I like honeydew melons. What about you?

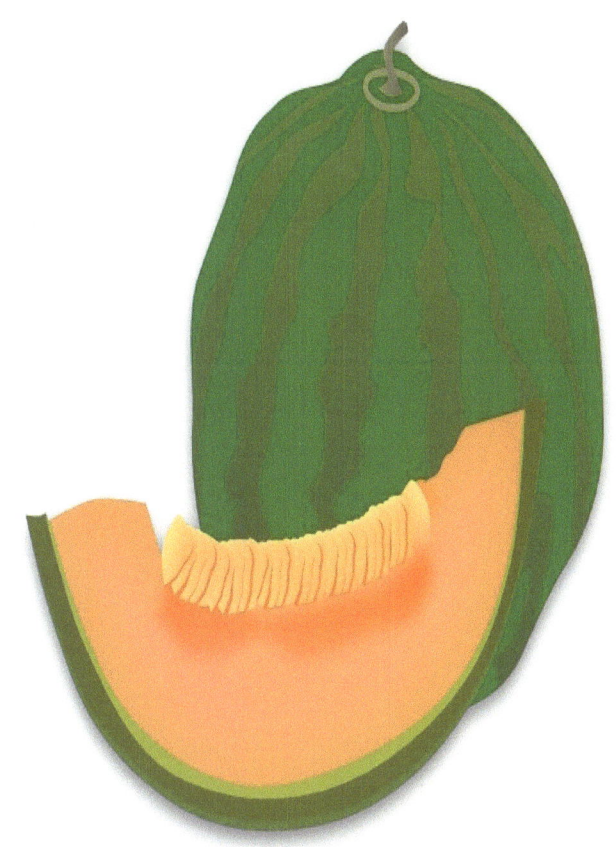

I like melons. What about you?

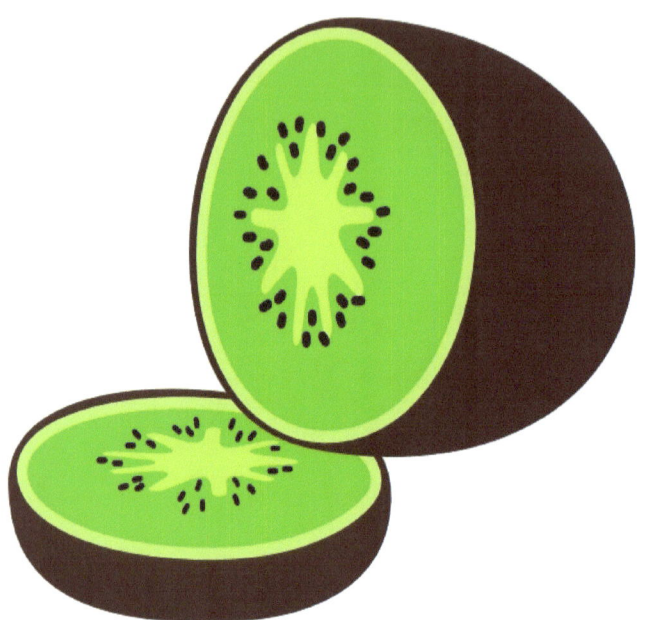

I like kiwi. What about you?

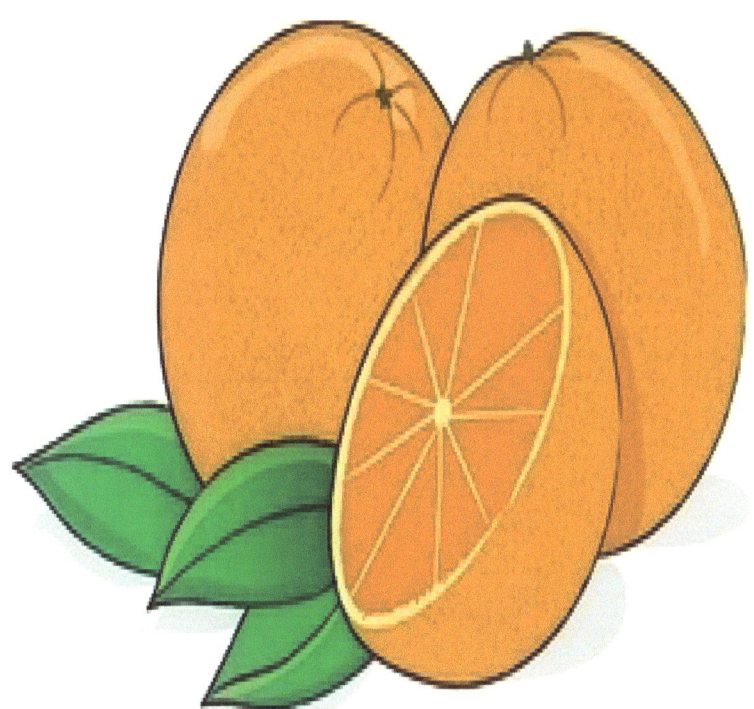

I like navel oranges. What about you?

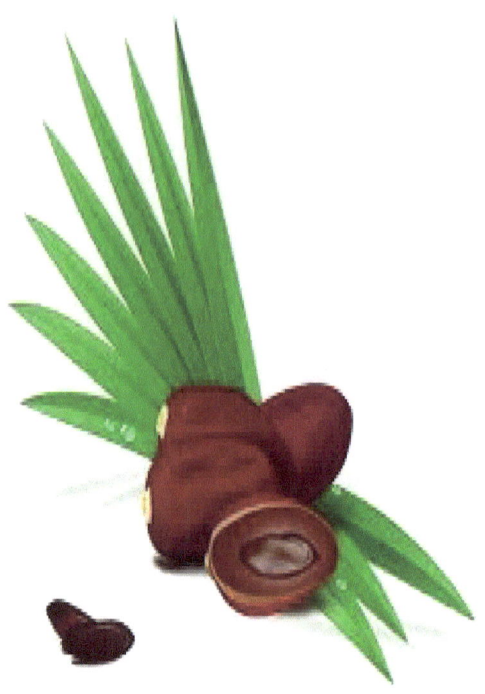

I like date fruit. What about you?

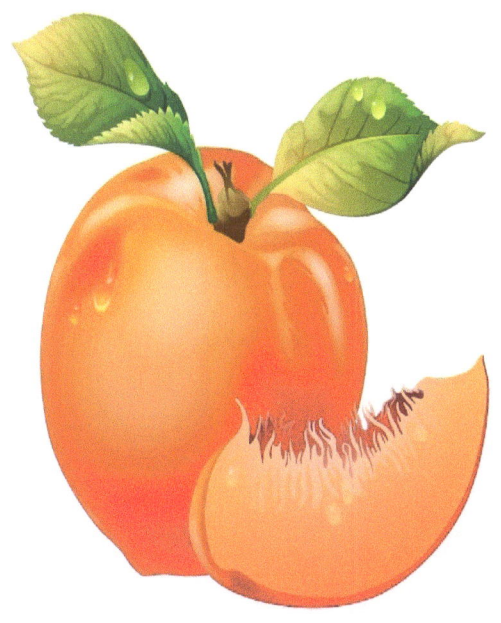

I like nectarine fruit. What about you?

www.ingramcontent.com/pod-product-compliance
Lightning Source LLC
Chambersburg PA
CBHW041533280526
45792CB00004B/1486